MEDICARE WARS:
Pamphlet 2
Stuff You Wish You Knew

Learn
Fight
Win

By
Charlene Brash Sorensen
Peggy Bechko

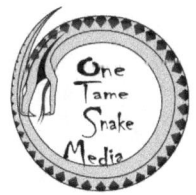

All rights reserved. No part of this book shall be reproduced, stored in a retrieval system, or transmitted by any means, electronic, mechanical, photocopying, recording, or otherwise, without the written permission of the publisher. The publisher and Authors assume no responsibility for errors or omissions. Nor is any liability assumed for damages resulting from the use of information contained herein.

This pamphlet contains the ideas and opinions of its Authors and is intended to provide informative and helpful material. This pamphlet is sold with the understanding that the Authors **are not engaged** in the rendering of professional services. For personal advice, the Authors recommend the reader consult a competent professional.

Copyright © 2017

This pamphlet is dedicated to Teddy Roosevelt who started a third political party, the Progressive Party (a.k.a. Bull Moose Party) in 1912. Roosevelt felt he could no longer support the direction the Republican Party was headed. Were you aware that as head of the Progressive (Bull Moose) Party, Teddy was the first President to come out in favor of universal health care as a right for all Americans? We came across this quote from a speech Teddy gave at Madison Square Garden a week before that 1912 election.

"The deliberate betrayal of its trust by the Republican Party, and the fatal incapacity of the Democratic Party to deal with the new issues of the new time, have compelled the people to forge a new instrument of government through which to give effect to their will in laws and institutions...Unhampered by tradition, uncorrupted by power, undismayed by the magnitude of the task, the new party offers itself as the instrument of the people to sweep away old abuses, to build a new and nobler commonwealth."

And, as to Social and Industrial Strength Teddy Roosevelt's party promised: *"The protection of home life against the hazards of sickness, irregular employment and old age through the adoption of a system of social insurance adapted to American use…".*

If you want to know more about Teddy's Progressive (Bull Moose) Party, here is a link to the 1912 platform. http://bit.ly/1912Progressive We urge our readers to read it, think about it, and consider how we can still aspire to those lofty heights.

Thank you Teddy for your inspiration to the Authors and for all manner of other inspiring thoughts.

Disclaimer: The information in this pamphlet is accurate to the best of the Authors knowledge upon its initial publication date.

In plain English: We are not responsible for any silly thing you might choose to do with information provided in this pamphlet.

Pamphlet 2 Medicare Wars Parts A & B

Table of Contents

Introduction	6
Original Medicare	9
Medigap Overview	29
Conclusion	59
End Pages	66

Introduction

Peggy: Well partner, it looks like we are ready to plunge further down the road of Medicare insurance. I think I understand how to enroll and how Medicare is funded. So now, I've got questions about what comes next. I know I get Part A automatically if I do blah, blah, blah… But, what happens after that?

Charlie: Let's start at the beginning once again and talk about what is known as "Original Medicare".

Peggy: Sounds good. Let's go. Maybe you can help educate us rookies on the details of Part A and Part B. You know, give us some ideas as to how to figure out what is best for us.

Charlie: One thing that needs to be clear by the end of this pamphlet is that the Medicare beneficiary is always seen as a source of "money". This is what our current system of turning health care into a business has done for us.

Peggy: So…you're telling me to "follow the money" again?

Charlie: It is ALWAYS the money.

Peggy: I want to know more than the dry facts. You know—who is doing what, how it works, those kinds of things. I'm getting kind of frustrated with all this and I admit I don't like just being a source of money in some "health care industry"! So the more I know, the better.

• • •

What's happening in the above exchange is an awakening on the part of one of the pamphlet writers (the not so Medicare experienced one) as to just how focused health care is on the making of money. It's an awakening that more people in the United States need to experience. The current design of "Original Medicare" is such that hospital and medical deductibles plus coinsurance costs result in a "gap" of full coverage.

For most people, Original Medicare will not be enough coverage. Insurance companies have stepped in to provide "insurance-on-insurance" to either fully or partially cover these gaps and they make plenty of money doing it.

The result of "Medigap" insurance coverage is that the senior (or disabled) persons with Medicare health insurance actually purchases insurance *twice*. If the "health care consumer" wants to purchase additional coverage, they must first pay the $134 per month (2017 Part B premium) and then select a "Medigap" insurer to cover the Part A deductible ($1,316 in 2017), the part B deductible ($183 in 2017), and some —or all— of the 20% co-insurance.

The first part of the pamphlet explains Original Medicare and the second part of the pamphlet talks in detail about "Medigap" insurance.

Original Medicare

What is Original Medicare?

Original Medicare is the term used to describe the combination of hospital coverage (Part A) and medical coverage (Part B) available to anyone eligible for Medicare health insurance coverage at age 65. We will talk in detail about coverage cost gaps in hospital and medical benefits and how they can be covered...or not. Remember... to purchase Medigap or Medicare Advantage (HMO) insurance you must first be covered under Original Medicare.

If you elect only to be covered by Original Medicare you can choose any participating doctor, hospital, or other provider *that accepts Medicare*. A Medicare "participating provider" is defined as follows:

*"Participating in the Medicare program simply means that the provider agrees to accept assignment for all services furnished to Medicare patients. By accepting assignment the provider agrees to accept the **amount approved by Medicare** as total payment for covered services."*

The following is a list of things that happen if your doctor, provider, or supplier accepts assignment:

- The provider agrees to charge you only the

Medicare deductible and coinsurance amount;
- The provider usually waits for Medicare to pay their share before asking you to pay your share;
- The provider has to submit your claim directly to Medicare and can't charge you for submitting the claim.

On the flip side…let's talk about those doctors (or suppliers) who ***don't*** accept assignment…

Non-participating providers have ***not*** signed an agreement to ***accept assignment*** for all Medicare-covered services. However, they can still choose to accept assignment for individual services. These providers are called "non-participating."

Here's what happens if your doctor, provider, or health care supplier ***does not*** accept assignment:

- You might have to pay the entire charge at the time of service. Your doctor, provider, or health care supplier is supposed to submit a claim to Medicare for any Medicare-covered services they provide to you;

- They can't charge you for submitting a claim. However, if they don't submit the Medicare claim once you ask them to, call 1.800.MEDICARE. In some cases, you might have to submit your own claim to Medicare using **Form CMS-1490S to get paid back;**
- The non-participating provider may charge more than the Medicare-approved amount, but there's a limit called "the limiting charge." The provider can charge up to 15% over the amount that Medicare approves. Non-participating providers are paid 95% of the Medicare fee schedule.

What the above discussion really means is you ONLY have access to those physicians and other medical providers who enroll to participate with Medicare. For example, where the Authors live only about 70% of licensed physicians in our town (Santa Fe, NM) accept Medicare assignment. In plain English, your choices are limited by the doctors' choice to participate with Medicare or not. Unless you have lots of money to go it on your own, your 'access' is **very** limited indeed.

It is important to pause a moment and talk about two of the biggest hurdles for Medicare enrollees. These are: (1) distribution of physicians who accept Medicare assignment and (2) the distribution of certain types of specialists.

With the majority of people on Medicare living in

Florida, Texas, Arizona and California this is where most specialists who routinely treat seniors are located. Once again we are forced to "follow the money". Really, since the practice of medicine is a "business" physicians will build their practice based on the location where they can make the most money. Can't blame them for behaving like businesspeople.

How about a real life example? One of the Authors just turned 65 and enrolled in Medicare. She lives in Santa Fe, New Mexico. As of April 5, 2017 there are NO Dermatologists in Santa Fe who accept Medicare assignment and also accept new patients. The closest Dermatologist accepting Medicare and new patients is in Albuquerque, New Mexico, which is about sixty miles south. The first available appointment is in September, 2017 — five months in the future.

Access my foot!

Let's Talk Original Medicare Coverage Gaps –

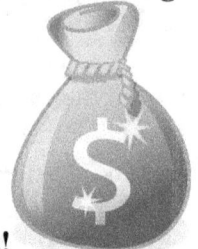

There are no free lunches!

Most people on Medicare ***don't pay*** a monthly premium for Part A (for more details see our first pamphlet in this series, *Medicare Wars, A Radical New Approach*). For those who don't qualify for the ***no cost*** Part A, they could pay a monthly premium that costs up to $413 per month if they paid Medicare taxes for less than 30 quarters (7 ½ years) of their working lives. If they paid Medicare taxes for 30 to 39 quarters (7 ½ to 9 3/4 years), the standard Part Amonthly premium is approximately $227 per month.

Remember: Medicare premiums can change every year - and usually do. Reality tells us with the current "health care is a business" system and multiple levels of administrative costs on top of spiraling medical costs, don't ever expect a downward adjustment to your premium.

Then there is that pesky hospital deductible of $1,316 for each *benefit period* (that's the current amount, it just increased in 2017 and could go up again in 2018). What the heck is a "*benefit period*"?

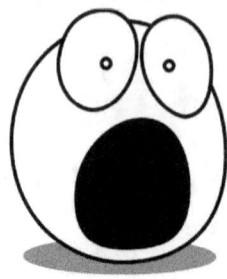

A *benefit period* is how Original Medicare measures the use of inpatient hospital and Skilled Nursing Facility (SNF) services. A benefit period **begins** the day you enter the hospital (or SNF). A benefit period **ends** when you have not received inpatient hospital (or skilled care in a SNF) for 60 days *in a row*.

In layman's terms–you are in the hospital for 21 days and are sent home. You pay your $1,316 deductible for that benefit period. Sixty-one days later, you are admitted to the hospital and (unfortunately) you now begin a brand new "benefit period" and a brand new $1,316 deductible you must pay as sixty days have passed since you were discharged.

The benefit period is **not tied** to the calendar year. There is **no limit** to the number of benefit periods you can have, or how long a benefit period can last.

For anyone with serious medical problems that could require several hospitalizations (and/or stays in a SNF), those deductibles could really add up! See below for an example:

Hospital Part A Deductible Example

Hospital Admission Date	Gap*	Hospital Discharge Date	Days in Hospital	Part A Deductible
January 1		January 22	21	$1,316
March 28	65 days	April 2	5	$1,136
October 1	153 days	October 10	9	$1,136

In the case of the table above, that's $3,948 in deductible charges in less than a year.

We would like to emphasize that there may well be additional costs with that $1316 deductible. For someone who is really sick not only will they pay the Part A deductible at the beginning of a benefit period but if they are in the hospital for longer than 60 days they will need to pay a **DAILY** coinsurance.

For days 61 to 90, the **DAILY** coinsurance is $329 **per day** and from day 91 and beyond that coinsurance goes up to $658 for each **"lifetime reserve day"**.

Let's give you an example:
- First inpatient stay is 70 days (days 1-60 at $0 coinsurance) but days 61 – 70 at $329/day. The

cost of this stay is the $1,316 deductible plus $2,961(co-insurance from you) for a total cost of $4,277;
- Sixty-one days later, this patient is admitted and stasy 82 days. The cost of the stay is the deductible of $1,316 plus 21 days at $329/day is $6,909 (co-insurance) or a total cost of $8,225 out of pocket;
- Total cost to the medical care "consumer" for those two stays is $12,502 out of pocket.

Let's think about this practically…

So the first hospital stay was an unexpected admission for pneumonia. The patient was very sick. Now the doctor wants to plan a scheduled hip replacement. A smart Medicare "consumer" would make sure the hip replacement happened within 60 days of the pneumonia discharge. No second deductible for this patient!

Peggy: But wait, back up…Exactly what are Lifetime Reserve Days?

Charlie: Let's see what we can do to make this clear —you know—"plain English" (which government and insurance companies are loathe to supply).

Original Medicare covers up to 90 days in a hospital for each "benefit period". We talked about this earlier in the pamphlet. In addition, each Medicare beneficiary has another 60 days of coverage (for lifetime reserve days). These days come with a big hitch—that is a very high coinsurance cost. Once these 60 days have been used, the Medicare beneficiary will be responsible for the ***entire cost*** of any hospital days beyond the 90 days for each "benefit period".

Examples are always helpful. Let us say you are in the hospital twice for 120 days during each benefit period. You would be able to use 30 of those lifetime reserve days for each stay. However, your "lifetime reserve days" would be exhausted—you know—GONE. You have none left for the remainder of your lifetime.

Let's provide another example related to cost…dollars out of **your** pocket. Presently most hospitalizations last less than a week. That's the good news. However, if you run into a situation like my friend did when his father was hospitalized for 136 days in 2010 that's a different story. Again, in 2016 his father had a similar lengthy hospital stay. His Medicare Part A (inpatient) out-of-pocket without a Medigap plan would have been $1,288 (2016 hospital deductible) for the first 60 days, $9,660 for the next 30 days, and $29,624 for the final 46 days. For a grand total of a horrifying $40,572.

But maybe you're one of those people who never get seriously ill and only need the occasional generic prescription for something minor. If that's the case you'll be fine with Original Medicare alone. Sadly, though, the past is not often a true predictor of what is to come. Who can predict with any certainty whether or not a catastrophic medical condition is just around the corner…or coming at some future date?

Most supplemental (Medigap) insurance policies pay all your hospital coinsurance costs plus up to 365 additional "lifetime reserve days". For many who have serious medical problems, this is reason enough to purchase supplemental insurance.

NOTE: You can always chose not to use your "lifetime reserve days" after you reach that 90 days in the hospital—if you want to save them for future hospital stays. That said, you would need to pay the higher hospital co-insurance ($658 per day in 2017) and let the hospital know "in writing" within 90 days of leaving the hospital. You would be totally responsible for these costs—or your insurer would — if you have one.

Yes, indeed, "health care insurance is complicated".

Similarly, if you qualify for a Medicare-covered Skilled Nursing Facility (SNF) stay, you will pay nothing for the first 20 days of your SNF stay within a benefit period. For days 21 to 100 there is a $164.50 coinsurance per day for each benefit period. After day 101 you pay ***all costs***. Those 60 lifetime reserve days apply to hospital PLUS SNF stays.

Medicare Part B Premium Increases

Before we complete the first part of the pamphlet and turn our attention to Medigap (supplemental) insurance, the Authors want to talk about 2017 Part B premium increases. The table below summarizes 2017 changes.

Who Pays What

	2013	2014	2015	2016	2017
Average	$104.90	$104.90	$104.90	$104.90	$109.00*
2016 New Enrollee				$121.80	$127.00**
2017 New Enrollee					$134.00***

*3.9% increase
**4.5% increase for 3 million who signed up for Part B for the first time in 2016
***23% increase for those who signed up for Part B in late 2016 or in 2017

The reason for the large Part B premium increase *for some* beneficiaries and not *for others* can be found in the Social Security Law - 1395r(f) hold-harmless clause. This provision limits the dollar increase for Part B premiums (physician services, outpatient hospital services, certain home health services, DME, etc.) to the dollar increase in an individual's Social Security benefit. Or...another way to say this...the payment for Medicare Part B premiums for individuals cannot rise faster than the benefits that individuals receive from Social Security.

NOTE: This does not prevent Medicare deductibles from also increasing (every year)—and by a *__lot__* more.

The *result of the rule* is that the net amount of a retiree's monthly Social Security check can never decrease due to rising Medicare Part B premiums.

What is truly weird about the "hold harmless" provision is that the rule was created to ensure that Social Security checks do not decline from one year to the next due to increases in Medicare Part B premiums. That said…If my Part B premium goes up by $5 in 2017 and my Social Security check goes up by $5 in 2017—I am STILL "running in place". I've received NO appreciable dollars in my Social Security check to offset inflation—except for one little part of my Original Medicare premium—Part B. And the Part B premium cost is not part of the formula used to determine Social Security cost of living increases. So, in TRUTH, I am still $5 in the hole.

Really? Does the government think that this card-shuffling trick is really going to work? Did YOU, our reader, just see what happened?

BUT – and this is a huge BUT – the hold harmless clause *does not protect* the following beneficiaries:

1. Those on Medicare do not receive Social Security benefits;
2. Those who enroll in Part B for the first time in 2017;
3. Those who are directly billed for Part B premiums;
4. Those who are dually eligible for Medicaid and the Part B premium is paid by the state; and
5. Those higher-income beneficiaries who pay income-adjusted premiums.

One point should be made here about those beneficiaries in #4 above—they will not see the impact of increased premiums but it DOES impact the state's Medicaid program which is "on the hook" for the increase.

To be included in the "protected" class of Medicare Part B recipients (you know, that 70% who didn't see an increase) the following would have needed to occur:

- The beneficiary was entitled to Social Security benefits in November and December of the previous year—2016;
- The Medicare Part B premium was deducted from the beneficiary's Social Security benefits from November 2016 through January 2017;
- The beneficiary does not already pay higher Part B premiums because of a higher income;
- The beneficiary does not receive a COLA large

enough to cover the increased premium.

Since the COLA for 2017 is NOT large enough to cover the *full amount* of the increased premium, if you are held harmless, your premium *does not* increase to $134.

Unfortunately, the remaining 30% of beneficiaries will pay most of the cost of the increase in Medicare premiums for 2017 for *all* beneficiaries. So…what this means in "plain English" is that this 23% increase for 30% of Medicare Part B beneficiaries reflects the true cost of the "official" inflation rate the Social Security COLA suggests. It is truly a Social Security 'pay cut' for new Medicare beneficiaries.

An Aside –

If you're turning 65 but you are not yet drawing Social Security you will receive the Medicare premium bill – Form CMS-500. This bill will be for a ninety day (one quarter…3 months) premium period. Medicare offers four methods to pay this bill:

1. Pay online through your bank website
2. Sign up for Medicare "Easy Pay"
3. Send a check or money order
4. By credit card

For information on Easy Pay, Google Medicare Easy Pay.

It is possible to pay on a monthly basis, but you will need to contact Social Security by phone to get information and arrangements. Social Security office phone number is 1-800-722-1213.

Skin In The Game

Peggy: I have a few things to say to Paul Ryan who claims that Medicare beneficiaries don't have any Skin In The Game.

I just can't let it go, I need to get my two cents worth in on this premium increase. I now realize if I had dropped my husband's insurance coverage in October 2016 my premium as a new Medicare recipient would have been $109 instead of $134.

I can't help it I have to rant because we are so being jerked around by our government. The folks in Congress apparently never check to see what's been in previous bills before they craft a new one, and I use the term 'craft' loosely because you have to question their intelligence and their sanity when you take the time to read some of the legislation that goes through.

Here's my latest scream. In our first pamphlet we stated what the government says, that 'most people' pay only $109 per month for Medicare and that, literally is true.

IF a person is already on Medicare the cost to him or her is $109 per month because, are you ready?, there is a 'hold harmless clause in a bill we read from back in another Medicare era. This clause states that the increase of Medicare premiums can never be MORE than the Social security benefit for that year. This is bad in so many ways it's hard to count and yet on the surface it may seem good. Here's how it works. If you're a person on $825 per month Social Security benefit, then in a way it's good since the increase can't be more than the increase in your Social Security payment. ***But wait! That means you get your Social Security cost of living increase wiped out by the increase of the Medicare premium you must pay. Ahhhh!***

Our government likes to pretend the cost of living went up by such a minuscule amount last year that the Social Security benefits rose only pennies and thus the Medicare Premium couldn't go up more than that. Really? Have they gone to a grocery store lately? Have they paid medical bills? Have they paid for gas, or utilities or local taxes? What about the Part B deductible that went up $17 in 2017 or the Part A deductible that went up $45 in 2017? Oh yeah, no hold harmless for the combined $62 Medicare deductible increases in just one year? So while they play their games and tell us they're not reducing our Social Security, they ARE, in a VERY big way. I'd like to believe they're unaware, but they're the ones who rigged the system, basing cost of living increases on such things as the cost of a new refrigerator, a computer and a TV when those aren't every day expenses and leading to a very false determination of cost of living. If they're that mean-spirited, we're in big trouble and voted poorly. If they're that stupid, we're in big trouble and voted poorly. Can we just throw them all out?

Charlie: This is truly messed up folks, I hope you are paying attention!

The rant is done…we're calming down. We'll go back to talking about Original Medicare costs.

Here we go again -- yet another calendar year deductible! More money that you must pay. The 2017 annual Part B deductible is $183 per year, up from $166 in 2016-a 9% increase in one year. Once you meet your deductible, you generally pay 20% of the Medicare-approved amount for the following type of services:

- Most physician services (including in the hospital);
- Outpatient therapy (physical therapy (PT)*, speech therapy (ST)*, occupational therapy (OT))**;
- Durable medical equipment.

*Medicare pays up to $1,980 per year (PT & ST)
**Medicare pays up to $1,980 per year (OT)

And here is a short list of some things Original Medicare *does not* pay for:
- 24-hour-a-day care at home
- Meals delivered to your home
- Homemaker services
- Personal care

Outpatient mental health services are covered under the Part B benefits with a 20% coinsurance including doctor and other mental health provider visits, hospital clinic/department, and some partial hospitalization services.

Outpatient hospital services (surgery center diagnostic

facility, etc.) also generally require a 20% coinsurance of the Medicare-approved amount for doctor/provider services. Don't forget…it costs more to get your care from a hospital outpatient setting than it would in your doctors office! You also might want to bear in mind that when in the hospital the Doctor can charge **every time** you're seen, even if he/she just sticks a head in to say hello, read your medical chart or does absolutely nothing. Now you can really appreciate that wonderful doctor pop-in where he says, "How are you doing?" and then runs for the door.

Wrap-Up

So, wrapping up the first section on Original Medicare the question arises: Is Original Medicare enough coverage without buying Medigap insurance or enrolling in a Medicare HMO? If you look at the numbers, **ONLY 14%** (2015) of Medicare recipients think the answer is "yes" because that is the number that have *no other coverage*. OR they simply can't afford to pay for any further coverage.

If you're feeling lucky OR you have a lot of money, you may feel that "Original Medicare" is plenty of coverage. But who among us can predict whether or not a very serious medical condition will happen to us at some time in the future?

Medigap Overview

Peggy: Oh boy! Look at the choices there are for Medigap insurance plans – 10 different plan types and in my zip code there are 44 different companies that offer at least some, if not most of these plans. I should be able to get a great deal. Take the edge off all those deductibles and coinsurance costs under Original Medicare. Competition helps bring costs down….right?

Charlie: Yes, there are going to be choices BUT they will be limited by the amount of money you have to spend—EACH MONTH on a premium. And don't forget those pesky annual premium increases. So we'll dive into whether it's worth paying for a Medigap insurance policy on top of insurance (your Medicare) when everything is taken into consideration.

Peggy: Oh come on! For cryin' out….I'm going to start screaming about planned bankruptcy again! Did you know that more than half the bankruptcies in the US are because of a medical calamity that hits a family? Okay, I want to keep screaming, but I guess we better get down to business.

Getting Down To Business

Medigap's name is derived from the idea that this type of additional private insurance covers the "gap" of deductibles and co-insurance that exists under "Original Medicare" Parts A (hospital) and B (medical).

The words "Medicare Supplement" and "Medigap" mean the exact same thing and the Authors will use them interchangeably.

As of year-end 2015, nearly 1 in 4 Medicare recipients were enrolled in private Medigap insurance. That's a whole lotta people!

Enrollment varies from 20-29% in the majority of the states (30) while in some states enrollment is as low as 3% (Hawaii) and in others as high as 51% (Nebraska). The highest Medigap enrollment is in the Midwest/plains states - above 40%. For those who are wondering (just like we did)...the percent of Medicare beneficiaries with Medigap plans has been stable since 2010, ranging from 27 percent to 30 percent each year. We *speculate* that this means only 27% of people on Medicare have enough discretionary income to pay the premiums for a Medigap plan which can be substantial.

The best time to buy a Medigap policy is the 6-month Initial Enrollment Period (IEP) that begins the first day of the month you are 65 or older ***and*** enrolled in Part B. An example would be, you turn 65 and are enrolled in Part B in June. Your six month Initial Enrollment Period for a Medigap policy is from June to November of that year.

After this enrollment period your option to buy a Medigap policy may be limited and it will cost more—unless you are in the "trial period". We talk more about the trial period later in this section.

NOTE: Even if you have health problems (pre-existing conditions) during the Medigap Initial Enrollment Period (IEP) you can buy ANY Medigap policy an insurance company sells ***for the same price*** as people who are in "good health". This is called Guarantee Issue. "Guarantee Issue" is when an insurance company is ***required by law*** to sell or offer you a supplemental (Medigap) policy **even if** you have health problems (pre-existing conditions).

If you chose a Medigap insurance plan when you turn 65 the insurance company **must** do the following:

1. Sell you a Medigap policy;

2. Cover all pre-existing conditions;
3. Not charge you more for the Medigap policy because you have past or present health problems.

NOTE: Removing the Guarantee Issue requirement is on the Medicare Reform Agenda of the current (2017) Speaker Of The House, Paul Ryan, and his fellow house Republicans.

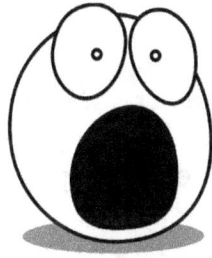

Okay, let's continue. Here are the seven additional circumstances in which Medigap insurance companies must provide you with "Guaranteed Issue" coverage:

Scenario #1:

You are enrolled in a Part C Plan (Medicare Advantage/HMO). The plan is leaving Medicare **or** stops offering plans in your area **or** you move out of the plan service area. You can enroll in any of the following plans sold in your state: A, B, C, F, K or L. You only have this right if you switch to Original Medicare rather than enrolling in another Medicare Advantage (HMO) plan.

You can apply as early as 60 calendar days before the date your Medicare Advantage coverage will end ***but no later*** than 63 calendar days after your coverage ends. Your Medigap coverage cannot begin until your Medicare Advantage plan coverage ends.

Scenario #2:

Your employer group health plan (retiree or COBRA) or union coverage that pays after Medicare pays is ending. You can enroll in any of the following plans sold in your state: A, B, C, F, K or L.

Here is the definition of COBRA from the U.S. Department of Labor:

"The Consolidated Omnibus Budget Reconciliation Act (COBRA) gives workers and their families who lose their health benefits the right to choose to continue group health benefits provided by their group health plan for limited periods of time under certain circumstances such as voluntary or involuntary job loss, reduction in the hours worked, transition between jobs, death, divorce, and other life events. Qualified individuals may be required to pay the entire premium

for coverage up to 102 percent of the cost to the plan.

COBRA generally requires that group health plans sponsored by employers with 20 or more employees in the prior year offer employees and their families the opportunity for a temporary extension of health coverage (called continuation coverage) in certain instances where coverage under the plan would otherwise end.

COBRA outlines how employees and family members may elect continuation coverage. It also requires employers and plans to provide notice."

You must apply ***no later*** than 63 calendar days after:

(1) the date your coverage ends,
(2) the date on the notice you receive that tells you that coverage is ending, or
(3) the date on a claim that is denied—if this is the only way you know your coverage has ended.

Scenario #3:

You have Original Medicare plus a Medicare SELECT (Medigap) policy and are moving out of the Medicare SELECT service area. You may keep your Medigap policy or switch to another Medigap policy. You can enroll in any of the following plans sold in your state:

A, B, C, F, K or L.

Here is a good definition of Medicare SELECT from *Go*Health:

"Medicare SELECT plans offer more affordable supplement coverage. How? SELECT plans negotiate with a provider network of doctors, hospitals, and specialists so they charge less for their medical services. These lower rates keep costs down for the SELECT plan provider, and plan members get lower premiums.

It's important to remember that plan members must receive their care from the provider network. Most of these networks include thousands of health care professionals, so finding a doctor or hospital near you usually isn't a problem.

Plan members will also need to get a referral from their Primary Care Physician in order for hospital or specialist care to be covered by the plan."

You can apply as early as 60 calendar days before the date your Medicare SELECT coverage will end ***but no later*** than 63 calendar days after your coverage ends.

Scenario #4:

You enrolled in a Medicare Advantage Plan (or

Programs for All-Inclusive Care for the Elderly) when you were first eligible for Medicare Part A (age 65). Within the first year you decide to switch to Original Medicare. You can enroll in *ANY* Medigap policy (A, B, C, F, K, L, M or N) sold in your state. This is called your "Trial Right" period.

Below is a rather lengthy (but we think important) explanation of the Medicare Advantage (HMO) "trial right" period.

You choose to enroll in an HMO but are worried that something might go wrong. Can you change your mind?

This is where the Medicare Advantage (HMO) "trial period" comes in—kind of like a "test run" for your new car. Medicare beneficiaries have a 12-month period to try out a Medicare Advantage plan. If you find that you are not satisfied, you can disenroll (drop out) of the HMO *anytime* during that 12-month period (prior to your one-year anniversary of the effective date). New Enrollees into Medicare Advantage plans need to be aware of this right because Medicare Advantage plans are not required to inform you at the time of your enrollment.

You are free to rejoin Original Medicare and you still have a "guaranteed issue right" to now buy a Medigap policy. The Medigap insurance company cannot deny you coverage—no matter what your health status is.

Here are the two situations in which this "trial period" applies:

(1) You joined a Medicare Advantage (HMO) plan when you were first eligible for Medicare at age 65;

(2) Beneficiaries who stay in a Medicare Advantage plan (HMO) for more than 12-months or have already used their one trial period can do one of the following:

(a) They can switch to Original Medicare during the fall Open Enrollment Period (October 15 – December 1) or

(b) The January Medicare Advantage Disenrollment Period.

NOTE: However, insurance companies offering a Medigap policy in most states can apply medical underwriting. The company can ***charge more***, or ***delay*** or ***deny*** coverage.

You can apply as early as 60 calendar days before the date your Medicare Advantage coverage will end ***but no later*** than 63 calendar days after your coverage ends.

Scenario #5:

You enrolled in a Medigap policy but dropped it to join a Medicare Advantage (HMO) plan or a Medicare SELECT plan for the first time. You have been in the Medicare Advantage or Medicare SELECT plan for less than a year. You want to switch back. You can rejoin the Medigap policy you were originally enrolled with if the same insurance company you had still sells your original policy OR if your former Medigap policy is no longer available you can buy a Medigap A, B, C, F, K or L plan. This is called your "Trial Right" period. (See definition under Scenario #4 above).

You can apply as early as 60 calendar days before the date your Medicare Advantage coverage will end ***but no later*** than 63 calendar days after your coverage ends.

Scenario #6:

You enrolled with a Medigap insurance company that goes bankrupt and lose your coverage. You can enroll in any of the following plans sold in your state: A, B, C, F, K or L.

You can apply no later than 63 calendar days from the date your coverage ends.

Scenario #7:

You leave a Medicare Advantage Plan or drop a Medigap policy because the company has broken the rules or you were misled. You can enroll in any of the following plans sold in your state: A, B, C, F, K or L.

You can apply no later than 63 calendar days from the date your coverage ends.

Please remember that different insurance companies may charge different premiums for the ***SAME EXACT*** set of benefits. As you shop around for a policy, be sure you are comparing the same policy. For example, compare Plan C from one insurance company with Plan C from another insurance company.

The "Alphabet Soup" of Medigap Insurance Plans

There are 10 standardized Medicare supplemental (Medigap) plans – A, B, C, D, F, G, K, L, M and N. There used to be E, H, I and J plans until 2010. Medicare enrollees who initially purchased one of these four (4) plans are allowed to continue their enrollment as long as they continue to pay their monthly premium. Medicare "claims" to have standardized these 10 plans back in 1990 in order to decrease confusion on the part of health care consumers when comparing coverage.

We say, "hahahahahaha."

Found below is a chart we created that compares the benefits and costs for each of those "alphabet soup" plans. It's so long you'll have to tip it sideways to read the chart.

Pamphlet 2 Medicare Wars Parts A & B

MEDIGAP PLAN COMPARISON TABLE

Basic Benefits	A	B	C	D	F**	G	K	L	M	N***
Hospital - Part A	Y	Y	Y	Y	Y	Y	Y	Y	Y	Y
Medical - Part B	Y	Y	Y	Y	Y	Y	Y	Y	Y	Y
Hospice - coinsurance & copayments	Y	Y	Y	Y	Y	Y	50%	75%	Y	Copayment Applies Y
Skilled Nursing	N	N	Y	Y	Y	Y	50%	75%	Y	Y
Part A Deductible	N	Y	Y	Y	Y	Y	50%	75%	50%	Y
Part B Deductible	N	N	Y	N	Y	N	N	N	N	N
Foreign Travel	N	N	80%	80%	80%	80%	N	N	80%	80%
Out-of-Pocket Limit*	N/A	N/A	N/A	N/A	N/A	N/A	$5120	$2560	N/A	N/A
Part B - Excess Charge	N	N	N	N	Y	Y	N	N	N	N

Y – Yes, Plan covers this benefit in full
N – No, Plan does not cover this benefit
N/A – Not Applicable

*After the Enrollee meets the out-of-pocket annual limit and the Medicare Part B deductible, the plan pays 100%

of Medicare-approved charges.

**Plan F offers a high-deductible option. This means the Enrollee pays for Medicare-covered costs up to the deductible amount of $2,200 (2017) before Medigap insurance pays. This chart does not reflect the high-deductible plan.

***Plan N pays 100% of the Part B coinsurance except for copayments of up to $20 for some office visits and up to a $50 copayment for an emergency room visit that does not result in a hospital admission.

NOTE: A copayment is a flat amount for medical services while a coinsurance is a percentage of the cost.

A Couple of Definitions

1. *Medicare B Excess Charges* are the difference between what the doctor charges and the Medicare approved amount. The doctor may charge up to 15% above the Medicare-approved charge.
2. *Foreign Travel Emergency* is a payment of 80% of the cost of ***emergency care*** during the first 2 months of each trip after the Enrollee pays a $250 deductible with a lifetime maximum of $50,000. For example, you are visiting Oaxaca, Mexico for the annual Day-of-the-Dead festival. You fall and break your wrist. The cost of your

care totals $5,000. For this you pay your $250 deductible and 20% of the remaining $4,750 for a total out-of-pocket cost of $1,200.

Exceptions

There are *always* exceptions to the rule. In Massachusetts, Minnesota and Wisconsin the basic Medicare benefits are standardized differently for Medigap from those noted in the Medigap Plan Comparrison Table. Sorry…if you live in one of these three states you will need to do some additional research!

Different Flavors of Alphabet Soup

The Author's discovered in their research that Congress passed a bill (HR2) on April 14, 2015 which eliminated plans that cover the Part B deductible for new Medicare beneficiaries beginning January 1, 2020. The only two plans that currently pay for the Part B deductible are Plans F and C (also the MOST popular Medigap plans). In 2015, nearly 6.5 million (or 55%) of all Medigap enrollees chose Plan F. Next in popularity were Plans N and C. On the other hand, while Plans K and L have pretty low premiums they only pay part (50% or 75%) of the cost of most Medicare coinsurances and deductibles. Once you reach a pretty big annual out-of-pocket maximum (currently under Plan K - $5,120) the Medigap policy then pays 100% of all costs.

Peggy: Man, plan K doesn't sound like much of a deal. So you are telling me that in addition to my monthly premium, I would be spending another $427 EACH MONTH if I divided that $5,120 deductible over 12 months?

Charlie: Yeah, you got it!

Congress believes eliminating first dollar coverage plans such as F and C will save Medicare money. This is hogwash and an attempt to deflect from the truth. The elimination of plans F and C, save insurance companies money — NOT Medicare. Medicare, after all, *never* paid the deductible—the enrollee was *always* responsible—unless they purchased a Medigap insurance plan that paid the Part B deductible. After this change, Medicare enrollees will only be able to choose a plan where they pay the Part B deductible not the insurance companies.

Who do these guys think they're fooling? Not our reader(s)! To quote the new head of CMS (Seema Verma) this type of change forces people to put more "skin-in-the-game". Isn't that nice!

The Author's would like to spend a little time sharing a bit more about the two newest Medigap plans – M and N.

Plan M – This plan has a slightly reduced monthly premium in exchange for the enrollees' willingness to pay *half* of the hospital deductible ($1316/$658) and *all* of the annual outpatient deductible ($183 – 2017). This Plan came into being with the Medicare Modernization Act of 2010. Current information shows that not many insurance companies offer this plan and not many people are enrolled; less than 0.5% of total Medigap enrollees in 2014.

Plan N – This supplemental option was created for health care consumers who like the idea of paying a lower premium in exchange for taking on a small annual deductible (it is the SAME deductible that everyone faces - $183) and some copays. In this case you pay no hospital deductible but you do pay the $183 Medicare Part B deductible and an office visit copayment of $20 per visit (primary care and specialty) and a $50 copayment for an emergency room visit. Current information shows that Plan N is offered by quite a number of insurance companies and is not very popular - 7% of all Medigap enrollees in 2014.

So let's get rid of the two most popular plans and create two new plans that nobody wants to purchase! So I want to choose either F Or C plan but the government wants to take away my choice and give me new choices *I don't want*. This one more time reveals the 'code word' problem with which they continually narrow the choices of the American public, all the while railing about 'choice'. So it boils down to THEIR choice, not YOUR choice.

Let us not miss the opportunity to confuse you further by including the Medicare SELECT option. This is available only in *some* states. Here is a good definition of Medicare SELECT from *Go*Health:

"Medicare SELECT plans offer more affordable supplement coverage. How? SELECT plans negotiate with a provider network of doctors, hospitals, and specialists so they charge less for their medical services. These lower rates keep costs down for the SELECT plan provider, and plan members get lower premiums.

It's important to remember that plan members must receive their care from the provider network. Most of these networks include thousands of health care professionals, so finding a doctor or hospital near you usually isn't a problem.

Plan members will also need to get a referral from their Primary Care Physician in order for hospital or specialist care to be covered by the plan."

The Authors say, "So, your 'choices' that everyone is always bellowing about are, once again, very much constrained." And, to our ears *SELECT* sounds an awful lot like a Medicare Advantage (HMO/PPO) plan. We will talk about HMO/PPO plans in our third pamphlet.

Time to Talk — Medigap Premium Costs

Cost varies based upon the specific "alphabet soup" (A, B, C, D, F, G, K, L, M or N) plan you choose *AND* the insurance company offering that plan *AND* your geographical location.

For instance, one of the Author's was comparing (for fun) Plan F here in Santa Fe, New Mexico and Plan F in Albany, New York. Wow…here in Santa Fe the monthly premium is $111.52 (Mutual of Omaha) while the same benefits in Albany, New York ranged from $187.75 (United HealthCare) to $449.76 (Bankers Conseco)! These rates were from February 2017.

Bear in mind that any of these premiums are *IN ADDITION* to your Part B Premium (average $134 – 2017). Costs may differ between insurance companies but the benefits remain the same.

Education Digression — Reading a Provider Statement

Pamphlet 2 Medicare Wars Parts A & B

The Authors are going to digress for a couple of pages and show the reader how to interpret a Provider Office Billing Statement.

Let us interpret the attached "Statement" below.

1. Beginning at the top is the "Payment Due" of $169.81. Where in the heck did this number come from?
2. The type of service this patient received is under the heading "procedure". This was an office/outpatient visit/new. This is a first visit by this patient to their new physician.
3. The physician charges $300 for a new patient visit. Currently the national average for a new patient visit is $330.
4. So what the heck is a write-off? This is the difference between what the provider billed Medicare and what Medicare actually *allows* for this service.
5. The patient balance is the amount that Medicare allows for this service. In the case of this patient, the visit is the first of the new year and they have not yet met their Medicare Part B deductible of $183.00.
6. The physicians charges $65.00 for a "complete" electrocardiogram.
7. This is the difference between what the provider billed Medicare and what Medicare actually *allows* for this service.

8. The patient balance is the amount that Medicare allows for this service - $15.72. In the case of this patient, they have not yet met their Medicare Part B deductible of $183.00.
9. The following are preventive services that have no charge – flu shot, pneumonia shot, calcium test, medication refill, tobacco survey, and pre-hypertension discussion.
10. Finally, "payment due" of $169.81 is the total of $154.09 and $15.72. Remember…this patient has not yet met their 2017 $183 Medicare Part B deductible. Therefore, they owe the entire amount to the practice.
11. This section identifies the provider as "accepting Medicare assignment". This is the place they would note if they do not accept Medicare assignment.

Pamphlet 2 Medicare Wars Parts A & B

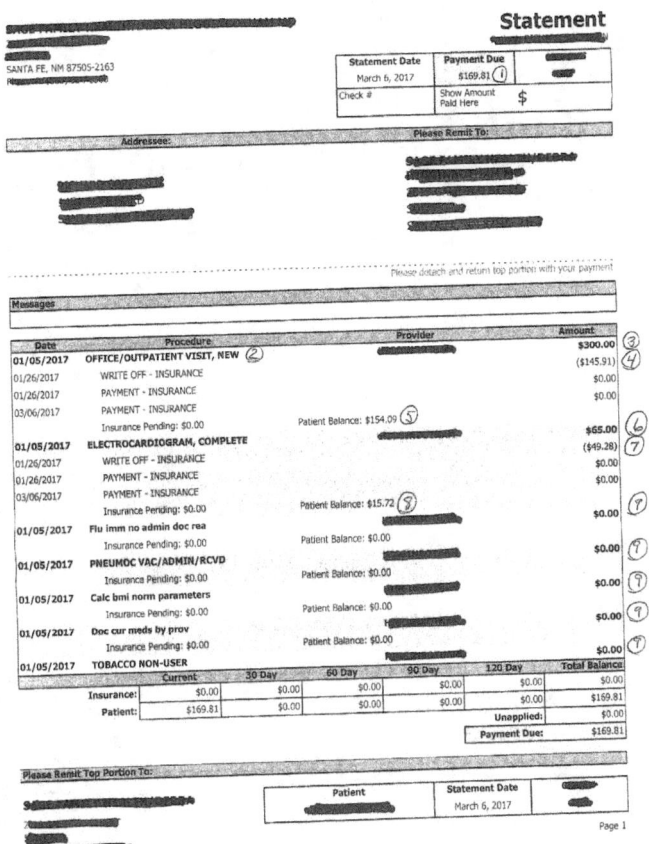

Pamphlet 2 Medicare Wars Parts A & B

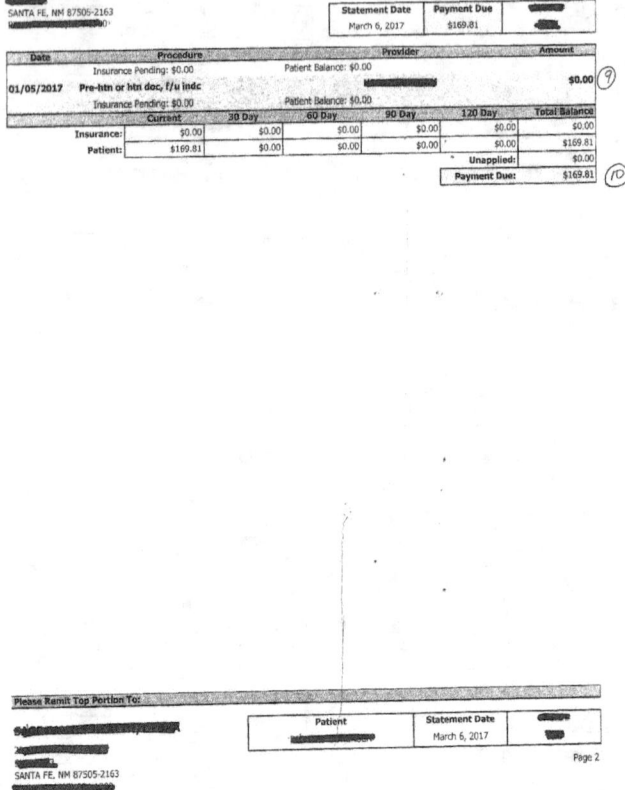

So what exactly is the provider "writing off"? They are writing off the difference between what they billed for their services -- $300 and $65 ($365 total) and what they were actually paid under the Medicare fee schedule. The Medicare allowable paid 54% of what the provided actually billed.

Four questions (we don't have an answer to):

1. Is the provider (i.e. doctor) "ripped off" by Medicare who only pays 54% of the billed amount?
2. Is the $365 billed by the provider the "true cost" of these services?
3. Is the "true cost" somewhere in between these two?
4. Is the amount paid by Medicare what these services are really worth?

As Trump said, *"Who knew health care was so complicated"*.

When Bernie Sanders (U.S. Senator from Vermont) was asked about this Trump quote by Anderson Cooper (CNN), Bernie said the following:

"Some of us who were sitting on the Health and Education Committee, who went to meeting after meeting after meeting, who heard from dozens of people, who stayed up night after night trying to figure out this thing, yeah, we got a clue," Sanders said. "When you provide healthcare in a nation of 320 million people, yeah, it is very, very complicated."

Stepping Back and a Bit of a Rant

Let us not forget that you are buying insurance on the insurance you already pay for! In fact you pay both the Medigap monthly premium which you pay directly to the insurance company PLUS your monthly Part B premium (deducted from your monthly Social Security check) and we have not even gotten to Part D (drug insurance) with the additional monthly premium you pay! Part D insurance is separate from Original Medicare and Medigap. As we mentioned briefly in Pamphlet #1, if you don't buy a Part D plan when you turn 65 you will have a lifetime late enrollment penalty.

Now for the brief rant...one question from the Authors is: Why do you still have to buy Part D coverage with the Medigap policy while most HMO/PPO (Heath Maintenance Organization/Preferred Provider Organization) policies include Part D coverage? We can't figure this out—it would be so much easier—you know, One Stop Shopping! Not to mention less confusion. But wait, it seems they want to keep us all confused. Yes, that must be it.

My writing partner is yelling about "going bankrupt" again. Time to calm her down with some green tea or maybe valium—if it is covered as a Tier 1 generic under her Part D (drug insurance) coverage—more on that

later... 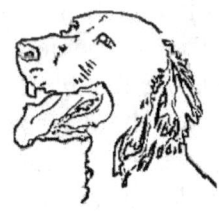 now let's all pet the doggie and calm down.

More Money Talk

We want to take a few minutes to discuss how Medigap insurance payments work with hospitals and physicians as opposed to the way health care claims are paid under the Original Medicare or Medicare Advantage Plans (HMO/PPO). We are going to need to talk about two different scenarios - one in which you have either Plan C or F where the $183 annual Part B deductible is paid or one in which you are responsible for the Part B deductible.

In the first scenario (the Part B deductible is paid under your Medigap plan), the physician sends their claim for your services directly to the insurance plan for payment. You have no out-of-pocket costs because your deductible is covered and you also do not have any responsibility for coinsurance.

In the second scenario (the Part B deductible is NOT paid under your Medigap plan), the physician will send their claim for your services directly to the insurance plan for payment. When the claim is 'denied" because you have not yet met the annual deductible for Part B ($183), the physician will send you a bill for your share of the cost. For more details, please see our previous example under "Reading a Providers Statement".

If your Medigap insurance does not pay the doctor directly, ask your doctor(s) if they "participate" in Medicare. This means they "accept assignment" for all Medicare patients. If the doctor does participate your Medigap insurance company must pay the doctor directly if you request. If they do not participate, the doctor may charge up to 15% more (*remember* excess charges) for their services and YOU would need to pay this difference. UNLESS, excess charges are a benefit as they are under plans F and G.

One of the most important goals to the Authors is education. So we are deliberately going to digress and talk about how doctors and hospitals are paid under Medicare.

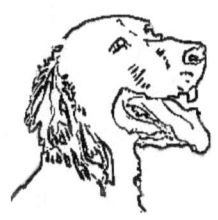

Education Digression — Paying Doctors and Hospitals

This is going to be boring—we admit—and this is going to be painful—we admit. Hang in there. Our readers really *really* need to "follow the money".

Medicare relies on a number of different approaches when determining how much to pay to each provider for services delivered to beneficiaries who have Medicare. Current payment systems have changed over time yet still are basically fee-for-service payments – in "plain English"…you get a Medicare service and it is paid.

Private insurers have generally designed their payment systems to match Original Medicare, that is, they pay for each service provided such as office visits, x-rays, etc. Again, each insurance company is duplicating an existing payment system. Remember those 44 different Medigap insurers in New Mexico (zip code 87505)? Well EACH of them duplicates the Medicare payment system. Every insurance company who pays for your medical costs will need to have the following type of staff: someone to enroll you, someone to answer your questions, someone to pay claims and someone to sell you their insurance. These layers of administrative costs get passed on to you in your premium.

Can you say-- administrative duplication and additional cost added to your premium?

Physicians and other health professionals: Medicare pays physicians and other health professionals (e.g., nurse practitioners) based on a fee-schedule that includes payments for over _7,000_ different listed services, i.e., new office visit, established patient visit, and shots. Rates are based on the *average costs* of providing health care services to a Medicare patient. They may be adjusted to account for other provider expenses such as malpractice insurance and office-based practice costs—you know, the new computer system.

Hospital Payments: The base rate for each hospital patient discharge is matched to one of over 700 different categories of diagnoses—called Diagnosis Related Groups (DRGs). DRGs that are more likely to require higher levels of care and/or more days in the hospital are assigned larger payments.

For example: a Patient is admitted with pneumonia as the diagnosis. The Patient has chronic heart failure. The discharge diagnosis (higher paying) is cronic heart failure with pneumonia.

Medicare's payments to hospitals also include money to pay for hospital capital (like a parking garage addition) and operating expenses—you know the costs related to labor—nursing staff. Some hospitals receive even more payments, such as teaching hospitals and hospitals that see more poor people who cannot pay for their hospital services.

Conclusion

Peggy: For God's sake Charlie for all we have done and researched ... what are they trying to do? Bankrupt us? It is confusing. It is expensive. Original Medicare was intended to eventually be for everyone beginning with those over age 65. Whatever happened to that simple plan? I remember my Grandfather...

Charlie: Yeah...remember when we figured out that Statement from a doctor's office?. Good grief...I think it took us most of an hour to decide exactly how much was owed for that visit. Complicated? Yes.

Peggy: Should it be this complicated? No.

Charlie: For me...the most shocking thing is really how ignorant I was about how much additional insurance to cover basic Original Medicare gaps really costs. Boy...I thought after 25 years in the "business" I was smart about this stuff. Wrong!

Peggy: It is simply outrageous that insurance is piled on top of insurance. You know...you buy the Medicare Part B for $134 a month just to help pay for medical costs. Then you buy Medigap coverage to pay for deductibles and coinsurance not covered under Part A or Part B. Then you have to buy that Part D to cover your drug coverage. And then you still don't have any dental or vision under Medigap. And why in the world is "vision" considered cosmetic? Eyes age...they go bad...you gotta read. What the heck? A Medigap plan? Yeah if you can afford one. Can I swear now?

Charlie: Well this is why we are going to do a third pamphlet because for those who cannot afford Medigap insurance coverage there is one *final* choice left—Part C, Medicare Advantage (HMO/PPO) coverage. Most Medicare Advantage plans include drug coverage

Peggy: Oh my gosh...is there more for my brain to absorb?

Charlie: To quote Trump, "....who knew health care was so complicated?"

Peggy: Bernie Sanders?

Charlie: Just finished reading "Our Revolution" by Bernie Sanders and my favorite paragraph from Chapter 4 – Health Care for All says it just this way:

"I have, for as far back as I can remember, always believed that health care is a *right* of all people, not a privilege. Health care is a basic human need. We all get born, we all get sick of have accidents, we all need care and die at the end of our lives. Everyone *needs* health care. Everyone should *have* health care."

Peggy: I also like what Al (Franken) has to say about universal health care:

"We need to go to universal health care as soon as possible…nearly half of all bankruptcies are caused by a medical crisis in the family. A single payer system would be the most effective in terms of reducing administrative costs, and I would be thrilled to support such a system. I would fight to make Medicare a true single-payer system."

The Wrap-Up

That just about wraps up this second pamphlet so I guess this is when we remind our Readers why we are writing and putting ourselves through the agony of trying to understand this "complicated" health care business.

So let's recap what Pamphlet #2 provides in education:.

- We explained what Original Medicare entails including the "basic benefits".
- We explained that Original Medicare actually has a lot of additional expenses beyond the "at no cost" Part A (hospital) including that really big hospital deductible of $1316, the $183 deductible for Part B (medical) and that pesky coinsurance of 20% for most medical services.

- We did not talk about any prescription medications because there is NO benefit for prescriptions under Original Medicare. (That comes in under Part D).

The second half of the pamphlet focused on explaining how Medigap (supplemental) insurance works and some examples of associated premium costs. The first line in every Economics textbook certainly applies here— There are no free lunches.

- We learned that there are 10 different types of Medigap plans offered by 44 (or more) different insurance companies in our zip code alone.
- We also learned that the current 10 types of plans ranged in monthly premiums from relatively low (meaning the plan pays for few of the financial gaps) to pretty expensive for full coverage.
- In reviewing these plan types it also become apparent that the premium differences by geographic area can be stunning—we shared some from Santa Fe, New Mexico where the Authors live to plans in Albany, New York— Wow!
- We also discovered that the monthly premium ranges wildly while still covering the *exact same* benefits. So it might cost me $100 bucks from one insurer for a Plan A package and $180 for a Plan A package from another insurer.

We are going to talk in some detail in our third pamphlet (Part C – Medicare Advantage - HMO/PPO) about how much duplication there is in administrative costs. Just think of those 44 different insurance companies who offer Medigap policies here in zip code 87505! ***Each one*** has enrollment, customer service, claims payment, and marketing administrative costs to pay for! Remember you are a CUSTOMER to the insurance company and a PATIENT and a CUSTOMER to the doctor.

Call to Action

CTA #1: If you have a Medigap plan, your CAT is to go scrounge around in your files (you do have a file we HOPE) and pull your policy. Look for the following:

- The Plan type (remember A, B,.......)
- See what your monthly premium is
- Determine if you pay for the Part A deductible
- Determine if you pay for the Part B deductible
- See whether you pay the 20% coinsurance or (if you have Plan N) the $20 copayment

Then add up your TOTAL monthly premium cost which would include:

1. Part B Medicare premium (roughly $134),
2. Medigap premium and any deductible that you

may pay. For example one of the Author's husband has plan A with a monthly premium of $129.
3. Her husband has to pay the $183 deductible before Medigap kicks in which would be another $12.20 per month.

So, in the case of her husband, his TRUE monthly costs are:

$134 – Medicare Part B
$129 – Plan A (Santa Fe, NM)
$12.20 – the Part B $183/year deductible distributed monthly
$34 - Part D monthly premium (this is prescription coverage)

Monthly out-of-pocket costs of: *$309.20*

If you had a hospital stay during the year, you would need to divide that $1316 by 12 to get a monthly premium to add to this total.

For those of you who really want to have fun. You can pull your supplemental policy from the previous year and compare premium prices from last year to this year. Did you get an increase?

CTA #2: From reading this pamphlet, do yourself a favor and begin reading AND saving every piece of information you get from your Medigap insurer and/or your doctor or other medical practitioner. But...before you file that away...we urge you to understand exactly what you are receiving. What we're saying here is you need to start paying attention.

If you do not understand what you have received, contact either the insurance company or the provider office and ASK until you "get it".

CTA #3: Pull your most recent physician and/or other health care practitioner "Statement" (remember the example from earlier in the pamphlet) and study and analyze it until you understand *exactly* what you are seeing. If you do not understand the Statement, we urge you to call and ask questions until you do "get it".

The truth is, you do have a choice. But there is a bind and that bind is in what you can afford to pay.

Choice #1 - Purchase Part B coverage... or not.
Choice #2 - You choose Part B coverage, now you decide whether or not to purchase supplemental insurance to cover the gaps of Original Medicare.

There is one last choice - Medicare Advantage (HMO/PPO coverage) which is the topic of our third in this series of pamphlets.

End Pages

This pamphlet is the second in a six Medicare Wars series. The first is currently available in paperback and Kindle editions:

Kindle & Paperback on Amazon:
http://bit.ly/MedicareWars1

The third pamphlet is currently in production and will cover how HMOs work with Medicare and more helpful tips and inside information.

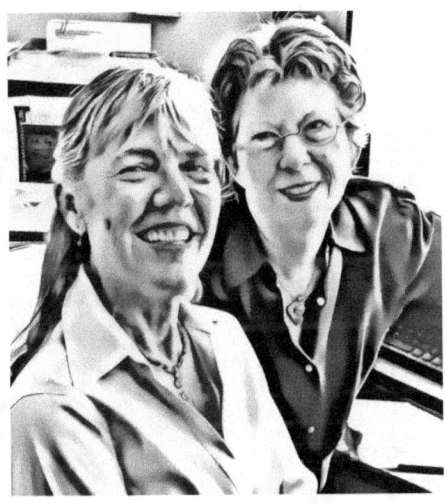

Charle: "Retired Health Care Executive"
Peggy: "Professional Writer"

www.ingramcontent.com/pod-product-compliance
Lightning Source LLC
Chambersburg PA
CBHW070719210526
45170CB00021B/1003